I0463533

Sleep Apnea Dream Killer

How A Sleep Disorder Nearly Devastated My Life

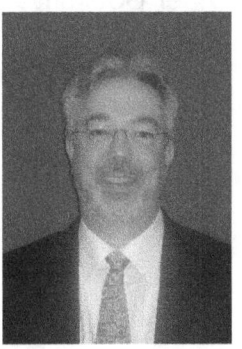

By David DeSchoolmeester

Copyright © 2014-2018 Your Authority Maker

TABLE OF CONTENTS

PREFACE:

According to the World Health Organization approximately 100 million people worldwide have Obstructive Sleep Apnea (OSA) (explained later in my story). In the United States, OSA is estimated to affect 1 in 4 men and 1 in 9 women; and affects 23 million working adults.

Approximately 4% of men and 2% of women over the age of 35 years have symptomatic moderate or severe OSA, affecting approximately 12 million people in the United States.[1, 2] It is estimated that less than 25% of OSA sufferers have been diagnosed.[3]

Therefore, we know that many people have the disorder and don't even know it. That's what happened to me for years. I had minor symptoms for several years (i.e. loud snoring, stop breathing for a second or two in my sleep, often wake up tired, etc.).

It was not until my symptoms became very severe and painful (wake up gasping for breath, severe and frequent migraine headaches, nearly falling asleep at the wheel of the car driving to work, etc.) that I had to find the cause and do something about it.

Many disorders, including Sleep Apnea, can be caused by another disorder; and vice-versa. Sleep Apnea is most common in obese men, but if these men were to lose the weight, it may be possible that it would go away. Chances are, this would only be the case if they did not have the disorder or any symptoms prior to gaining the weight that made them obese. Two thirds of men & women in America are overweight, fat, or obese. With the U.S. population more than 314 million people (July 2011 US Census Bureau), there are an incredible number of people who potentially have Sleep Apnea.

I, however, was not the usual case; I was diagnosed in my 30's while I was still a very thin man. So, most likely, when I lose the weight that has caused me to be obese, I would probably still have Sleep Apnea. Although, I am sure it would be less severe and more easily controlled.

Many patients who have sleep disorders often have other health issues. While, it's hard to say what came first; for instance I have severe Sleep Apnea, Depression, Obesity, Diabetes and High Blood Pressure; this is not uncommon. They are all interrelated. My diabetes did not start until after I was 48 years old and obese (at the time I already had all of the other health issues).

It is very likely that when I bring my weight down to a more healthy level for my height and age, the Type II Diabetes will go away. More than likely the High Blood Pressure will drop off as well; the depression and the Sleep Apnea will lessen in severity due to being healthier overall.

It is easy to see why many countries that have government controlled health care strongly encourage individuals to join wellness groups to exercise, lose weight and reduce or eliminate unhealthy practices. In fact, physicians in Italy, France & Germany receive bonuses for signing up more patients to these wellness programs (Documentary, "Sicko", by Michael Moore).

The rest of this eBook is my story of very severe Sleep Apnea that became out of control for three years. I had been on Continuous Positive Air Pressure – CPAP (explained later) therapy treatments for the disorder for more than 12 years before it became uncontrollable. It took three years for the doctors to identify my problem and get it under control. As my story unfolds, I will describe the incredible series of events that transpired and how my life was nearly taken from me. It is my hope that you read my story and get something of value from it for you, your family or a friend.

Most of what we learn in life comes from either personal experience or networking (learning from others personal experiences). With the sizeable number of potential Sleep Apnea sufferers, the chances are good that you either live with or know someone with the disorder. I know more than 15 people through work, family & friends (outside of my research). Everyone needs to read this!

DISCLAIMER:

I am not a Medical Doctor, Nurse Practitioner, Nurse or even a Pulmonary Technologist. I am just a patient who was originally diagnosed in September 1997 and has been treated for Sleep Apnea ever since.

As I am not a medical professional, I am not giving any advice, nor should you take it from me or anyone that is not a medical professional. By reading this eBook, you automatically agree not to hold me liable in any way to any ailment you may have.

DEFINITIONS:

First, let's define a few terms you will hear about in this book. These initial definitions are from Dictionary.com

Alzheimer's disease:

Often shortened to: Alzheimer's, it is a disorder of the brain resulting in a progressive decline in intellectual and physical abilities and eventual dementia. Named after A. Alzheimer (1864 – 1915), a German physician who first identified it.

Dementia:

A deterioration of intellectual faculties, such as memory, concentration, and judgment, sometimes accompanied by emotional disturbance and personality changes. It is caused by organic damage to the brain (as in Alzheimer's disease) or by head trauma, metabolic disorders, or the presence of a tumor.

Diabetes:

1. Any of several disorders characterized by increased urine production

2. Also called diabe-tes mel-li-tus, a disorder of carbohydrate metabolism, usually occurring in genetically predisposed individuals, characterized by inadequate production or utilization of insulin and resulting in excessive amounts of glucose in the blood and urine, excessive thirst, weight loss, and in some cases progressive destruction of small blood vessels leading to such complications as infections and gangrene of the limbs or blindness.

3. Also called Type I diabetes, insulin-dependent diabetes, juvenile diabetes. A severe form of diabetes mellitus in which insulin production by the beta cells of the pancreas is impaired, usually resulting in dependence on externally administered insulin, the onset of the disease typically occurring before the age of 25.

4. Also called Type II diabetes, non-insulin-dependent diabetes, adult-onset diabetes, maturity-onset diabetes, a mild, sometimes asymptomatic form of diabetes mellitus characterized by diminished tissue sensitivity to insulin and sometimes by impaired beta cell function, exacerbated by obesity and often treatable by diet and exercise.

5. Also called diabe-tes in-sip-i-dus, increased urine production caused by inadequate secretion of vasopressin by the pituitary gland.

Heart Attack:

Damage to an area of the heart muscle that is deprived of oxygen, usually due to blockage of a diseased coronary artery, typically accompanied by chest pain radiating down one or both arms, the severity of the attack varying with the extent and location of the damage.

Hypertension / High Blood Pressure:

Arterial disease in which chronic high blood pressure is the primary symptom.

Sleep Disorder:

A disturbance of the normal sleep pattern

Apnea / Sleep Apnea:

A temporary suspension of breathing,

occurring in some newborns (infant apnea) and

in some adults during sleep (sleep apnea)

Hypopnea:

Abnormally shallow breathing, usually

accompanied by a decrease in the breathing

rate

Central Sleep Apnea (CSA) – from WebMD:

CSA occurs when you temporarily stop trying

to breathe because your brain briefly does not

signal you body to do so. It is most common in

overweight men over 40. Breathing is disrupted regularly during sleep because of the way the brain functions. It is not that you cannot breathe (which is the case for Obstructive Sleep Apnea); rather, you do not try to breathe at all. The brain does not tell your muscles to breathe. It is usually associated with serious illness, especially an illness in which the lower brainstem – which controls breathing – is affected. In infants, it produces pauses in breathing that can last 20 seconds.

Obstructive Sleep Apnea (OSA) – from WebMD:

OSA occurs when you regularly stop breathing for 10 seconds or longer during sleep from an obstruction in the nose, mouth or throat. This

usually occurs when the throat muscles and
tongue relax during sleep and partially or
completely block the airway. Other factors that
make sleep apnea more likely include using
certain medicines or alcohol before bed,
sleeping on your back, and being obese.

Stroke:

1. A sudden severe attack, as of paralysis or
sunstroke

2. A sudden loss of brain function caused by a
blockage or rupture of a blood vessel to the brain,
characterized by loss of muscular control,
diminution or loss of sensation or consciousness,
dizziness, slurred speech or other symptoms that

vary with the extent and severity of the damage to

the brain

MY STORY:

Sleep Apnea is just now beginning to come out of the closet to be known by the masses as something worth taking note of. Ever since NFL Superstar Reggie White died on December 26, 2004 from complications caused by the Sleep Disorder, Sleep Apnea, the world has started to realize how much sleep disorders can affect your health. But the affects don't stop at merely your health, as if that was not bad enough!

Many people, especially over weight middle-aged men, may have a sleep disorder and not even recognize it as a problem. Some just say, "Well I snore a lot, but what does that have to do with anything?" That could mean the difference between life and death! It's time for everyone to realize this and report problems, no matter how minor, to their healthcare professional. Early detection is the key to proper treatment and reducing potential damage to your body and overall health.

I was way outside the normal or average candidate parameters for Sleep Apnea when I was diagnosed in 1997. I was a thin, tall, young man of 36 years old. Prior to being diagnosed, I was suffering from frequent and severe Migraine Headaches. I came very close to losing my job for taking so much time off from work.

I went to the doctor immediately upon experiencing the first Migraine Headache because the pain was so excruciating I could not stand it. Up until that point, I had never experienced such severe pain in my life. When it came on, I had to be in a quiet room, lying down with the lights off and a warm compress on my forehead and eyes.

My doctor began to treat the symptom of my headaches and also began testing to determine the root cause so that it can be treated. Because of my thin structure, his thoughts did not even consider Sleep Apnea. We looked at the potential for allergies, changes in living conditions, and possible sinus issues. None of them were a problem and the migraines kept on the attack.

Finally, he began asking questions of my wife about many things, including how I slept. She had stated that for many years now I was having breathing issues in my sleep, but neither of us thought much of them at the time. I had these all the way back to 1991, yet the sleep disturbances my wife described were becoming more frequent and more disturbing. She explained that she noticed I would stop breathing periodically throughout the night, mostly for just a few seconds, but sometimes for much more!

In September of 1997 I was given my first diagnostic sleep exam. It is performed in a clinic where you go to sleep for the night, during which time you have approximately 25+ electrodes/wires attached to your body to monitor an enormous amount of information. While you sleep, you are monitored for events like:

- Changes in your breathing
- Snoring, amount & how loud
- Other physical obstructions to your sleep
- Heart rate
- Eye movements
- Leg movements
- Tossing and turning
- Oxygen levels in your blood stream
- Depth of your sleep
- And much more

It's absolutely incredible, how much information is captured during your sleep at the clinic. The main characteristics that we needed to know were:

- How many times did I stop breathing,

- For how long each time and

- What were my oxygen levels throughout the night?

In the 5 hours that I slept at the clinic, I stopped breathing 83 times! These ranged from just 2 seconds to well over 2 minutes in length. During which time my blood oxygen levels dropped well below the normal range.

The Sleep Doctor told me I had Obstructive Sleep Apnea and needed to be put on a CPAP machine. Remember this was 1997 so, like most people at the time, I had no idea what that was or what it meant. He told me there are two main types of Sleep Apnea:

1) Obstructive

2) Central

Remember, Obstructive Sleep Apnea (OSA) events are caused by a physical obstruction in the throat or neck area that "obstructs" or impedes your breathing; and Central Sleep Apnea (CSA) events occur when your brain forgets to tell your body to breathe.

He went on further to explain that a Continuous Positive Air Pressure device or "CPAP" is used to keep a positive air pressure in my respiratory system while I slept. I am to wear a mask that just covers my nose and is attached to a six (6) foot hose that comes from the CPAP machine on my night stand next to my bed. There are other masks as large as one that covers your nose and mouth, but I could not use one like that since I am a "belly-sleeper". This machine will be set at a specific pressure so that it will keep my airway open while I sleep, preventing the occurrence of or minimizing the effects of apnea events.

I didn't particularly care for the idea of wearing such a device while I slept, but I gave it a try. The very next morning after the first use, I awoke feeling much better. I realized that I had previously been very tired and my thoughts seemed as though my mind were in a fog. Then after sleeping with this device for just one night, I felt like I could think more clearly, I felt like a big veil had been lifted from my mind; and my body felt refreshed. I actually dreamed that night. It was only then that I realized I had not had a dream for more than a year. I felt more energized and ready to take on the new day.

Until you have this type of miraculous change take place in your life, you don't realize how bad off you really were. Sleep Apnea, like many disorders, does not just come on you all at once. It usually begins and builds so slowly in your life that you hardly recognize the minute changes happening every night. Until one day:

- Your spouse complains about your snoring;
- You put on some weight and begin to feel more tired and less rested every day;
- You start to fall asleep on the couch after a normal days work;
- You have no energy to do things around the house or go out anymore;
- You begin to have unexplained headaches that take longer to go away than usual;
- It becomes harder to concentrate at work and at home;

- You miss important deadlines at work;

- You miss important dates at home;

- You get diagnosed with other illnesses like high blood pressure or even diabetes;

- You feel depressed all of the time;

- You don't feel you have the strength to make it through the day;

- You even begin to wonder why you bother getting out of bed each morning;

- And you may get so bad as to contemplate ending your life.

I know, I've been there; and it is not something I want to go through again!

Many of the symptoms I just mentioned could be misdiagnosed very easily as simple Depression, Chronic Fatigue Syndrome, Early signs of Dementia, Early signs of Alzheimer's Disease, etcetera.

Sleep Disorders, like many other medical problems, can have very serious effects on your body as a whole. This is not the type of thing that you can die from directly; because eventually your body will take that next breathe. However, they weaken your immune system, can cause you to become less active and it becomes the root cause of all kinds of physical and mental issues that will arise or worsen. For example:

Your Sleep Apnea causes you to be overtired and therefore, less active; decreasing your desire to exercise; your bad cholesterol goes up or your blood pressure goes up OR BOTH! You are then a good candidate for a heart attack or stroke, and guess what? You have a heart attack or stroke and die.

Sleep Disorders wear you down and cause other health issues to arise or magnify. I know by my own experience. In February of 2008, I had routine Diagnostic Sleep Test performed. In March of the same year, I accepted a new position that required me to move my family from South Florida to the New Orleans area. When I arrived in Louisiana, I mentioned to my new physician that I had a sleep test performed, but did not receive the results. I asked her to review my test results and let me know if there was anything to be concerned about.

I went on about my new job, found a new home and moved my family. A few months later, I began feeling noticeably tired throughout the day and just passed it off as "new job jitters". It did not take long before I began missing deadlines, not getting back to people on important issues and not being able to handle the amount of work I was given. A few more months went by before this began to be noticed by some of my coworkers; and more importantly, my boss.

I began to be very concerned and went back to the doctor. One year after my last diagnostic sleep test, I had another doctor print out the sleep report so that I can review it myself. It indicated two items of real concern:

1) I had ZERO - 0% REM sleep (REM stands for Rapid Eye Movement – but more importantly, it is the point where you enter deep restful sleep, also the point at which you would normally begin to dream) and

2) A medication I was taking had been indicated as one that might inhibit proper sleep.

I immediately took action to get all of my medications evaluated for potential side effects and ended up having two of them changed. I also went to a sleep doctor to see about changing my air pressure and getting my Sleep Apnea under control.

I had already started to gain weight and having other health issues like hypertension; depression had set in, worrying about my job; and I was having tremendous concentration and memory issues. I was exhausted each night after a normal day at the office.

Because of my memory and concentration problems, I was then given a Neuro-Psychiatric Evaluation; where your memory is tested for 5 to 6 hours. The exam has you matching/recognizing faces, pictures and shapes; repeat sentences spoken to you; make shapes from blocks; etcetera. An example of one of the test modules has two 3" x 4" spiral notebooks, each containing 50 pages. The first notebook had one picture per page. You carefully examined the pictures on each page. Then you went to the second book where there were two pictures per page. One image was in the previous notebook and one was not. You then had to determine which image, of the two, were from the first book. About 2-1/2 hours later you would return to the second book to see how many images you could get right after more time has past.

I received scores from the Neuro-Psych exam that were below the normal range and discussions of early dementia or Alzheimer's disease began with my doctor. Caused by the Sleep Apnea, the memory and concentration problems I was experiencing could be temporary or permanent. At this point there was no way of knowing. This started to scare me tremendously; which only accelerated my depression and changed my eating habits to appease my depression.

Before long, I could not do my job, not even the most basic aspects of it. I was so depressed; I came home every night and sat in my chair watching TV all night long. I stopped doing work around the house, like cutting the grass, and many nights barely even spoke to my wife and daughter. Because of my poor job performance, my boss ended up giving me three choices to choose from:

1) I am fired;

2) I take a Disability Retirement; or

3) I take a voluntary reduction in pay to a different job where she had an opening.

I could not stand the idea of being unemployed, so I took the voluntary reduction in pay losing $22,000 in annual salary (approximately 25% of my salary). Plus, I thought that if I can beat this things that was causing all of this to happen, that it would be harder for me to re-enter Federal Service if I took the Disability Retirement. It was also very embarrassing for me coming to work each day with the same people looking at me like I am a broken-down shell of a man. Whether that was actually on their minds or not, my own negative feelings of self worth were making me feel that way.

My boss arranged for me to do my new job at home. It was performed almost entirely online, so that was an option I was afforded and I took it.

I kept going back to the sleep doctor, getting air pressure changes to my CPAP and unfortunately, not getting any better. My wife began to doubt my ability to make rational decisions at home or handle the budget. When I looked into her eyes, I did not see a loving caring sole anymore, but rather a scared individual who began to distance herself from me. My daughter, sixteen years old, began to doubt my ability to give her the guidance that she had grown accustomed to and needed from her father.

I now began to have a hard time doing my new job. I had numerous air pressure changes and three more sleep tests in just two years. It was not long before I was required to go back to work at the office, due to job performance issues working from home. Coming in each day and seeing the same faces, mostly just ignoring me and barely giving me any notice, made me very uneasy at the office. I suppose they did that so they did not have to talk to me. I felt shunned by a couple of people; who at one time were my peers as well as friends and I was treated indifferently by the rest.

My depression continued to worsen, I did nothing but go to work, come home, go to bed and go to work again. Even on weekends, I never left the security of my chair in the Family Room. Change after change in air pressure (I lost count after 19) and nothing worked to make things better.

After months of working to improve my job performance, my boss sat me down and told me that I was going to be put on a Personal Improvement Plan (PIP). I knew this was done to show a paper trail in the event I cannot perform adequately, they can show that every effort was extended to me and I failed. Then they would be able to fire me and withstand any backlash, should I try to get a lawyer to fight it. I was now making $22,000 less than when I was in the position I came to New Orleans to fill and had been for quite some time. The only saving grace is that I did not purchase a home that would have required my previous pay to keep. Like everything else in my life at the time, I failed the PIP.

At the same time I had been fighting the relocation company, which my employer hired, over a contract dispute to a guaranteed home purchase benefit I was supposed to have. We lost our South Florida home to foreclosure and took a 100+ point hit on all three of our credit scores. This has been an ugly fight in that my employer completely backed out of having any responsibility. I felt betrayed by my employer and of the relocation company.

My depression had become so severe that all I could think about was how inescapable my situation had become. I had lost all respect from my workmates, my family and myself. I believed that it was only going to continue to worsen, until I would not remember how to drive a car or even feed myself. I felt the world had come crashing down on me and it was not letting up. A tremendous flood of dark emotions kept creeping in, wave after wave, until I finally threw my hands up and asked God to take my life. He refused and some small sense of Christian belief left in me would not allow me to take my own life. I had thought very seriously about it, but in my mind I kept seeing the loving eyes of my daughter and it was that love that prevented me from taking action to end my existence.

Finally, in December of 2010, my sleep doctor had discussed a newer therapy with me that he wanted to try. This was the last thing he had to offer me and said if this does not work, he has nothing else. It was called BiPAP with AutoSV for complicated sleep disorders. BiPAP, means there are two pressure settings "Bi" Positive Air Pressure "PAP" and AutoSV stands for Automatic Servo Ventilation; which is a pressure support ventilation automatically delivered as soon as my breathing drops under a certain flow value for a specified amount of time. My Sleep Apnea had morphed into a very complex type consisting of both Obstructive AND Central Sleep

Apnea events. This new type of therapy is designed to catch intermittent breathing and make it more regular.

For me, this is how it works: There is a higher pressure setting for when I am breathing in to open my airway completely; when I breathe out, the machine switches to a lower pressure (still keeping the airway open, but allowing me to exhale); then a timer starts and if I do not take another breathe within a couple seconds (approximately 2) the machine will force me to inhale at the higher pressure. This now has a pressure high enough to prevent obstructions and regulates my breathing should my brain forget to tell my body to breath.

The therapy is working! I began feeling much better and thinking more clearly within a couple of days. After six weeks on the new machine, I went back into the doctor for him to pull the data off the computer chip in the machine that is monitoring my sleep. I went from an average of 35 Central Sleep Apnea events per night (before the new machine) to only 8 per night. The doctor stated that I may have some permanent damage and may not be able to get back to the level I was years earlier, and that it will take some time before we know for sure.

The good news was too late for my life at home. The stress and strain of the Sleep Apnea, Type II Diabetes, High Blood Pressure, Obesity, Depression along with the financial issues had finally broken my wife as she announced she was leaving me. The drama of the last three (3) years was too much for her to continue. Even as I had given her the good news that the therapy was working, she already had an apartment and moved out.

The good news was too late for my work life as well. My boss had to take action on a failure in my job and at the PIP I had been placed on months earlier.

So, again, I was given my pick of three (3) choices:

1) I am fired;

2) I apply for disability retirement or

3) I voluntarily take a reduction in pay (AGAIN) to a position she had available.

Again, I chose to stay employed, hoping that with the new therapy I am on, I can prove that I am better and move back up the "Corporate Ladder" (so-to-speak) I spent the last three (3) years falling down. This new job came with an additional $11,000 per year decrease in pay.

So, in three years I had lost $33,000 in annual salary, my marriage, my health and my career to

Sleep Apnea. The changes in my health over the last three years were so debilitating, I now have to take a handful of pills every day and closely monitor my blood pressure and blood sugar. I have high blood pressure and I was just diagnosed with diabetes. In the last three years I gained 65 more pounds and I am on anti-depressant medication.

All of this happened to me over the course of just three (3) years. Fortunately, I kept after my healthcare providers to resolve my problems. Believe it or not, I consider myself lucky. Especially when I think what would have happened if I did not keep after my health issues to resolve them! I know I would have broken through those Christian values and very possibly would have taken my own life, if I did not die from complications of Sleep Apnea first.

But today, I am feeling better, I have more control over my thoughts and I am dreaming again (both in my sleep and for the future). I have more energy to get my fat butt off the couch and start exercising. Even though there is no chance of reconciliation with my wife, I have maintained a friendly relationship with her and I now live for my children.

I am beginning to piece my life back together again..........

I have started a Social Media Marketing business (Seaside Web Solutions; www.seasidewebs.com), *forgive the plug*, to replace my job. Pronounced "J" "O" "B"; the nastiest 3-letter word I know.

I am beginning to regain by employer's trust again and have started to successfully take on more responsibilities. As I prove myself, I am given additional tasks that are increasingly more difficult.

So far, that has not coincided with an increase in pay, but I know the request has been made by my supervisor.

This does not mean that I will recover to the level of ability that I was 3-1/2 years ago. I may and then I may not. In February of 2011, I had another Neuro-Psychological examination. This time the result was much better. All of my scores were in the "normal" range; the low end of normal, but normal just the same.

I do not think I will ever get back to the level I was in 1997 before I was first diagnosed with Sleep Apnea. In my twenties, I was in the United States Navy Nuclear Power Program; a very intense and highly technical field. Given the circumstances for which I have been put through, I do not think I will recover to that level of effectiveness.

This saddens me greatly. Although, I am better than I was more than two (2) years ago and I am still progressing. It is very hard going to work day in and day out with people that watched me fail.

I thank God every day for the miracles he has worked in my life and the testimony he has given me. I lost a wife, $33,000 in annual salary, my credit, and numerous other things, including the trust of my peers. But God saved me from ending my life; allowed me to survive and to tell my story so that others can benefit.

He is replacing the things that were taken from me. I am now dating a wonderful Christian woman and I have resurgence in a business that I enjoy. It is my hopes that I will someday replace my J O B with this business and help as many other people as I possibly can.

It is my dream that this book reaches out to those who are suffering and gives you hope for recovery. I wrote this eBook to shed light on how deeply a sleep disorder can affect your life and health. Take this to heart, in the spirit it was written.

Sleep disorders can have an enormously devastating effect on your life and health if you do not do something about them. I have a friend that has been diagnosed with Sleep Apnea, has a CPAP therapy machine at home and does not use it. For all of those people out there...........take my advice before it's too late! Get help and **USE your CPAP / BiPAP / BiPAP-AutoSV device as prescribed**!

Okay, I didn't want to do this, but you forced me. From an online article, here are some scary numbers:

"The statistics surrounding sleep apnea deaths are alarming. About 14.6 people per 1,000 die from sleep apnea each year. According to national research, nearly 40 million Americans who are at risk for obstructive sleep apnea death go undiagnosed. Almost 1,400 traffic deaths occur annually because people who suffer with sleep apnea are driving tired. About 17 percent of the population has sleep apnea and the greatest risk group is male between the ages of 40 and 70." [4]

Does this scare you? Well, it scares me! This is nothing to play around with. If you wake up tired, snore excessively, wake yourself up gasping for breath or your spouse tells you that you stop breathing briefly while you sleep…………GET YOURSELF TESTED!

Don't play around with your life! You may have less of it left than you think!

I wish you all well and may God Bless you.

David DeSchoolmeester

REFERENCES:

1. Young T, Palta M, Dempsey J, et al. The occurrence of sleep-disordered breathing among middle-aged adults. *New England Journal of Medicine 1993; 328; 1230-1235.*

2. http://www.census.gov

3. http://www.apnexmedical.com/downloads/Apnex_Medical_OSA_FAQs.pdf

4. http://www.sleep-insomnia.net/death-from-sleep-apnea/

Brought to you by Your Authority Maker @

www.YourAuthorityMaker.com

OTHER BOOKS BY DAVID DESCHOOLMEESTER

Below is a list of other Business and Non-Business books I have written. All are available on Amazon Kindle via the links provided…

Business:

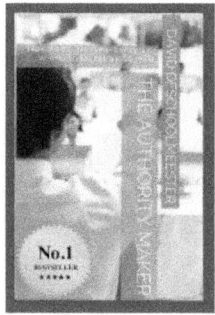

The Authority Maker

Be The One Everyone Wants To Do Business With

(https://www.createspace.com/5009225)

- We all know that everyone wants to do business with the "One that Wrote The Book". Having Authority in a particular subject pulls in prospects and potential customers/clients/patients. This book will not only teach you the importance of Authority, but how to build it quickly to grow your business or practice. It is built on methodologies learned from several expert Internet Marketers like Frank Kern, Mike Koenigs and Dan Kennedy.

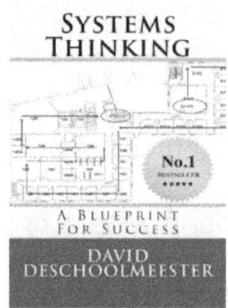

Systems Thinking A Blueprint For Success
(https://www.createspace.com/5001918)

This book discusses the great need for

systematizing your business NOW! Small

Business owners have really taken a hit in the last

decade and this book will take a look at why and

what the small business owner should do about it.

Follow the most successful business model in the

world!

Reinvent Yourself And Survive Today's Economy

(http://www.amazon.com/dp/B007HB8HGY)

- Throughout my working life I have had to "Reinvent" myself many times, for one reason or another. In this book, I discuss those reinventions and how to go about doing it for yourself to give yourself a new fresh start. You may be forced into it, due to the economy and corporate downsizing, but there is a way to help yourself through it.

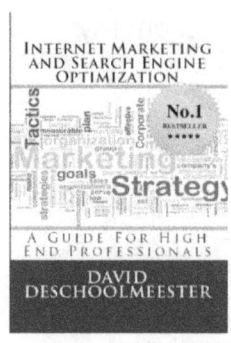

Internet Marketing And Search Engine Optimization –

A Guide For High-end Professionals

(https://www.createspace.com/5019986)

- This book is a very short guide designed to education busy professionals, like Lawyers, Physicians, Surgeons, Dentists, etc. You are way too busy to have to learn how to market and advertise your practice on your own, but today that is just what many of you need to do. This book will help to teach you some things you need to know in order to hire the right person to promote your practice like it should be promoted.

Non-Business

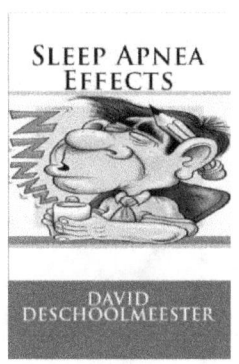

Sleep Apnea Effects

(https://www.createspace.com/4989907)

- I performed a great deal of research for this book. It lists all kinds of affects that Sleep Apnea has on your body. Does Sleep Apnea kill? Not directly, but there are numerous ways in which it can indirectly – the kind of things you'd be a fool to disregard. Also inside this book are the transcripts of an Interview I had with the Head of Pulmonology at Tulane University School of Medicine and Sleep Lab.

www.ingramcontent.com/pod-product-compliance
Lightning Source LLC
Chambersburg PA
CBHW051250170526
45165CB00004B/1646